The Leverage Diet

The Answer to Weight Loss for Emotional
Overeaters and Chronic Dieters

Rachel E. Short

Disclaimer

Always consult with your physician before beginning any diet or exercise program. This book is not intended to diagnose or treat any physical or emotional health condition or disease.

Dedication

To my husband Mick, you are my true love and the brightest star in my universe. You inspire me with your determination and the ferocity in which you pursue your dreams. You are an action-packed trail blazer, a man larger than life, and I will love you for the rest of my life.

To Mom, Dad, and my sister Sarah, you are my heart and soul for all time.

To all my family and friends, I love you and wish you happiness and peace in this life we share together.

To everyone on the planet, be good to each other and to the animals.

Thank you to Dafeenah at Indie Designz for your phenomenal creations of cover art and website.
http://www.indiedesignz.com

Thank you to author Lizzy Ford and the great IT Sherpa Matt from the Guerrilla Wordfare team for your guidance and help, I couldn't have done this in any way without you.
http://www.guerrillawordfare.com.

CONTENTS

My Mission

I will present The Leverage Diet for the world to read. Those that will benefit from this book have a similar history of weight problems and failed dieting as I have. Anyone that has repeatedly tried and failed diets can benefit from this book.

Do you have trouble losing weight? Are you depressed about your weight? Maybe you have been struggling for years. You've failed so many diets it's not funny anymore. Your physical and emotional health suffer because you can't lose weight. Dieting just seems too hard. You are frustrated, tired of "feeling fat", and desperate to lose weight.

Maybe you overeat to make yourself feel better or to help you manage your stress. Maybe there are other reasons. As a result, your body has grown bigger and your health has declined. You may be caught in a vicious cycle of feeling bad about yourself, overeating to feel better, gaining more weight, then feeling worse. Finding a way out can seem hopeless.

But it's not hopeless. I found a way out of this self-destructive cycle, by chance, or maybe by destiny. The resolution came to me in the form of The Leverage Diet. With this book, I sincerely hope to help you escape the suffering you have endured and propel you to a new level of living after successfully losing the weight that has plagued you for so long. I hope for you to finally be free.

Introduction

The purpose of this book is to share with you a method I stumbled upon that helped me stick to a diet long enough to lose weight. The Leverage Diet is *not* another fad diet, magic weight loss pill, or quirky diet and exercise program. If you've been dieting as long as I have, you are probably aware of the hundreds of different weight loss products and programs already out there. And, if you're like me, you and I are part of what has made that weight loss industry a multi-billion dollar market, yet you are probably still stuck being overweight and miserable.

The concept of Leverage Diet is not new, complicated, expensive, or secretive. It's actually pretty simple, and pristinely effective. I have been dieting for over 15 years That's over 50% of my life at this point in time. I have been *unsuccessfully* dieting for 100% of those years, and have gone through periods of extreme emotional overeating, binge eating, poor self-esteem, and depression about my weight. When I created and followed The Leverage Diet, I was 100% successful the very first time. In fact, it worked so well that I began writing this book before I was even finished with the program. That is how confident and excited I am about this and why I want to share this with you.

I realize that not everything works for everyone, but my hopes are that this diet method will work for you so that you can finally break your emotional overeating and chronic dieting cycle, and stick to a diet long enough to lose that weight.

Chapter One

Inside the Mind of a
Chronic Dieter and Emotional Eater

I consider myself a chronic dieter. The term "chronic" refers to on-going, long term, or frequent. In between bouts of stuffing my belly with as much food as it would hold, I started a new diet at least 15-20 times a year while I was struggling with my weight as a teen and young adult. My diets usually started on a Monday. I breezed through the first day on the diet, possibly the second day, but by the third day I started to panic. Because I no longer received the inside-out hugs from an overstuffed belly, I felt a painful loss.

Hunger pangs felt like full blown emergencies, and I was desperate to make those raw, gnawing feelings go away by again eating as much food as I could hold.

Short-lived diets may have resulted in 2-3 pounds lost at the most, but I could never stay on them long enough to lose more weight. Many times after a failed diet attempt I overate to the point where I actually gained a few pounds. Desperation overtook me early into the diet and I began missing the highs the food gave me. I couldn't stand to be without those highs. Failed diet after failed diet got me nowhere except feeling even worse about my weight, then overeating to feel better, only to gain more weight. The self-destructive cycle had an iron grip on me.

I came out of high school weighing about 160 pounds at a height of 5' 3-3/4". I had been overweight since I was at least 10 years old. One of my early childhood memories regarding my weight was around the time when the movie Batman came out, the one with Michael Keaton and Kim Basinger. In one scene, Batman was preparing to hoist himself and Vicki Vale up the side of a building, and Batman asked Vicki (Kim Basinger) how much she weighed. Her answer was "about 108." I remember thinking to myself, "W*ow, I better not gain anymore weight, because I'm already 110 pounds and I'm only in fifth grade. So, I better not eat too much from now on.*"

Looking back, I realize that I used food to cope with the social anxiety and depression I encountered as a child and teenager. I was an "emotional eater" and I overate to soothe negative emotions and stress. Food was always there for me, my go-to medication for feeling stressed, hurt, and exhausted.

As a child, I was referred to as "shy." That meant I wasn't very talkative to people other than my parents and my sister. I was quiet and well behaved in public, as my parents would confirm if asked. If memory serves me correct, the first sign of what I would eventually call "social anxiety" showed up when I was in fifth grade. The first days of school are always hard for kids. Everything is new: new classroom, new teacher, new subjects, and a new group of classmates.

I remember lunch time on the first day of fifth grade. We were lead single-file into the school kitchen to pick up a tray and go through the lunch line, the cafeteria workers putting together our lunch as we slowly walked by. That part wasn't so bad, and the fact that we were told to stay in our line as we left the kitchen to sit down at the lunch tables wasn't so bad either. But the walk to the lunch table unveiled for the first time an enormous cafeteria with a vast ocean of noisy, unfamiliar kids. I felt each pair of eyes on me, burning me... watching me like sharks watch helpless little fish swim for their lives before they dart in for the kill. I held my breath during the entire painful walk to the table, my body tense and my walk hurried and awkward.

I didn't know the girl to my right, the boy in front of me, or anyone at the long rectangular table when it was my turn to sit down. To my relief, to my left was a wall, a merciful wall that wasn't going to look at me or talk to me. If I could have disappeared into that wall, I would have. That happy, peaceful, inanimate wall was the only relief I would feel until lunch time was over.

I began eating. I don't remember what it was, but it was the school lunch of the day. I mostly kept my eyes down, staring at the food while I tried to eat it without being messy. And without realizing it, with every bite, I covered my mouth with my left hand as I chewed. I was painfully aware of the strangers at my table, sitting uncomfortably close to me. At one point, I glanced up to see the boy in front of me kind of laughing at me. He said with a smile, "You don't like anyone to see you chew, do you?" I was appalled. Someone was talking to me? Oh my gosh. I shook my head no and managed a half-smile at the boy, but that was all. I ate slower after that, silently begging time to hurry up so lunch would be over.

My "shyness" worsened as I got older and moved up in school grades. My early teenage years brought exponentially more uncomfortable scenarios, mostly because those years were heavily concerned with what social circles we all were in. The kids were bigger, meaner, and the social pressures much heavier. I longed for the easy fifth grade days where even though I had to sit by strangers, we were all assigned a place to sit and we didn't have to worry about having friends to be able to sit at a table to eat. I had some "friends" at school that I hung out with just to make sure I had somewhere to sit at lunch time, and someone to stand around pointlessly with at recess. Although I would rather have been alone, I knew I had to group up with someone just to survive the social seas. There were a lot more sharks in the junior high and high school waters than there ever were in fifth grade.

High school. Being in large groups of people was even more excruciating, and if I could have skipped lunch time I definitely would have. In class I usually sat in the back to limit the number of shark eyes that could see me at one time. Even though I was in the back of the class, I sat with my head on either hand to try to cover up my nose because I was embarrassed about it being too long and pointy. Talking in front of the class when answering a teacher's question or when I had to make a mandatory presentation was torture for me. I sweated, shook, and my face turned beet red every time. I could hear my heart beat in my breath when I talked, I only hoped no one else could.

Not only was I struggling with my then undiagnosed "social anxiety," but I was also overweight. Being a fat teenager added even more anguish to my daily life and it made my social status even worse. The "popular" girls in school were all thin and were years ahead of me in their makeup and clothing. My weight had been slowly creeping up since junior high and in high school I considered myself fat and ugly. Boys weren't interested in me and I was kind of glad, I didn't want anyone talking to me no matter who they were.

Due to my "shyness" and emotional sensitivity, I developed the keen ability to hear teasing, taunts, and mean jokes from other kids, whether whispered in class or belted out at feeding time. Their cruel words and fat jokes always seemed to be directed at me, although they rarely ever were. I was too smart, quiet, and unassuming to be a target of bullying. As a quiet kid and a good listener, I picked up on more belittling and berating comments than I ever cared to hear.

I did encounter several minor instances of kids making fun of me for being overweight, both girls and boys. But I wasn't the fattest girl in school and I stayed out of sight as much as possible so I didn't have to face the wrath of the meanest situations or bullying. I witnessed other girls and boys get hounded almost daily for being overweight or for some other shallow reason bullies create to make a sport out of torturing others. Some of the nicest kids were pulverized by emotional and physical bullying just because of their weight or appearance.

In one high school incident, as I was walking through the hallways between classes I happened to pass by the gymnasium. There was a small crowd of kids peeking in the gym, so naturally I went over to see what they were looking at. Much to my horror, I saw a girl I knew laying on her back on the floor, and two other girls standing over her hitting her and wagging their fingers in her face, saying "stay down there you fat b****".

The scene was gruesome to me. I was enraged. I daydreamed about charging over to the bullies and knocking them down to help the poor girl on the floor. But, being the "good kid" that I was, and feeling afraid of any disciplinary consequences I would face, plus the retaliation that would certainly come from the bullies in the future, I did nothing.

To this day, I think about that girl on the floor, and I wish I had acted differently. The bullies didn't like her because she was heavy and was also a little slow mentally. I took her suffering personally, and I've carried it with me ever since, my inaction weighing heavily on my mind.

My diet habits in the junior high and high school days consisted of cereal in the mornings and a packed lunch that my wonderful mother made for me daily. Dinner would be of her making as well. My main meals were fairly healthy, but it was all the snacking I did at home while no one was around that added pounds.

At home after school, when no one was looking, I gobbled down peanut butter and brown sugar sandwiches, sometimes twice a day. They were extremely high in calories, fat, and sugar. Another favorite of mine was a piece of bread with butter, micro-waved to melt the butter, and then topped with table sugar. A couple of those and a Coke or Pepsi would satiate my cravings and soothe me from all the chaos I went through at school. I was always glad to get home, away from the social pressures, but just being home wasn't enough, I had to self-soothe with food in order to regain my peace of mind. Unfortunately, my peace of mind came at a great cost. The very habit I developed to make myself feel better was the culprit behind my being overweight which only made my teenage life harder.

After high school, I went straight to college and lived on campus. Within my first year, I gained 15 pounds and tipped the scales at 175. The "Freshman 15" came true for me. There was an abundant supply of food on the college campus, which only made it easier for me to overeat. During this time, my parents were going through a divorce and my sister - my only sibling and lifelong best friend - was thousands of miles away serving in the military. She was struggling to adjust to her new life in the Army and had to make great emotional and physical sacrifices to do so. She had always been there for me, a year and a half my senior, and I never had to be truly alone or without a friend. But she was unreachable. I couldn't help her, she couldn't help me. When she left for the military, the "rug" was pulled out from under me, and a part of me will never get back up from that.

Mom and Dad were struggling with their new found status of "Divorced", each trying to cope and make sense of life. Living separately after nearly 18 years of marriage, they both had their own demons to fight, and new hopes to grow. Our family was broken and we were all trying to deal with the painful emotions that came with our new life situations.

Our torn family life became the driving force behind my emotional overeating. I felt lonely, empty, broken, and hopeless. Food was my way of self-medicating. I ate as much as I could, carelessly, at every meal. My full stomach simulated an inside-out hug, the physical pressure actually providing a sense of comfort.

My first two years of college presented me with two facts. First, I felt emptier and lonelier than ever, living away from the home that I still couldn't believe had broken apart. And second, I had access to unlimited foods and meal times on campus. Those two factors accelerated my emotional overeating habits and left me at 175 pounds by the end of my sophomore year. Luckily I was able to find the best group of friends possible for me at the time. They were smart, responsible, and stayed up late doing their homework instead of partying. They were a source of strength for me, albeit temporary.

I met a guy and transferred to a college in New York for my Junior and Senior years in college. The 600 mile distance between me and the scene of my broken family helped me suppress the feelings a bit, but I was still very depressed and battling the same social anxiety that had followed me everywhere since my youth. And I had no idea that I was in for another life-altering event in my new Long Island life, one that would make my parents' divorce seem petty.

I was finishing up my final semester at the end of 2001. Up until this time period, I had been maintaining my weight at 175 pounds. But in the fall of 2001 I became the primary caretaker of the "guy" behind my 600 mile move. We got engaged shortly after September 11, the fateful historical day filled with both fear and heroism. My then- fiancé was dying of cancer. The cancer had been eating away at his spine and he slowly lost the ability to walk and care for himself. At the age of 21, I faced end-of-life issues that most people don't have to deal with until they are older.

Due to the extreme emotional stress of the situation, I didn't have the emotional or physical energy to feed myself and I mostly stopped eating altogether. There were some days that the only meal I ate during the day was a bag of chips and a Coke from the vending machine on my college campus. Over the course of a few months, this was all I could manage for myself and my weight plummeted by 40 pounds.

My then-fiancé had been gradually losing his appetite and the need to eat due to the ravenous effects of the growing cancer and his declining health. This combined with the sheer terror of the situation and the lack of energy to feed myself left me unable to properly care for myself.

While this is a sad part of the story, take heed, there is useful evidence about dieting and weight loss here. Weight loss occurs as the result of eating less than normal. I lost weight by eating less than normal, even though it wasn't an intentional or healthy method.

My 40 pound weight loss and the emotional trauma of the experience left me feeling weak and unwell for several years. I moved back home with my mother a year after the death. My mother and other family members couldn't believe how thin I was. She would hold up her index finger and say, *"This is what you look like. You look like a walking bone."* I think it scared her to see me that thin, and it was beginning to scare me as well. So, I started eating again.

By the time I married my husband Mick in 2005 I weighed 155 pounds. I felt healthy and fit at that weight, and my family said I looked healthy and fit. I felt the same and thought it was probably going to be a good target weight for me. Unfortunately, I did not stay at that weight for long. It wasn't two years later that I began tipping the scales at 175 again.

As an adult in my twenties, I didn't have to face pressures from the narrow social setting of my school days, and I felt some relief from that. But my social anxieties weren't limited to school and being a teenager. I continued to experience social anxiety in many situations although I had learned to work through it a little better than I used to. Stopping at a gas station to fuel up my car was always an event (and still is!). First off, if I wasn't feeling brave enough at a particular time to pull into a station and be viewable to the public eye, I wouldn't stop at all. And If I *really* had to get fuel, and the fuel gauge was on "holy cow!", I found the most comfortable feeling gas station and did what I had to do. The situation would still leave me stressed out and anxious, even though I didn't talk to anyone. Just the thought of going somewhere new, with people around that could look at me with their shark eyes, was enough to press my social anxiety button.

The consequence of having my social anxiety button pushed was usually going home to stuff my belly with too much food. The driving force behind my emotional eating shifted from social pressures at school, depression over my parents' divorce, and the experience of a death, to the everyday life pressures of a maturing adult still struggling with social anxiety.

Sometime in 2008, I developed a chronic bingeing habit. I had a 50+ mile commute to work and sit at my desk for nine hours, resulting in almost 12 hours a day of being sedentary. Sitting all day has never felt good to me. A car accident in 2005 left me with chronic neck and back pain, and the sedentary lifestyle I had only compounded it. To help me cope with the relentless aches and pains and the daily stress, after a work day I habitually stuffed my stomach full of food until it hurt. Strangely, the pain in my belly had a satisfying effect, because it took the focus away from my neck and back pain and the emotional stress I was struggling with and diverted my attention to the actual physical pain in my stomach.

My daily stresses as a maturing adult were pretty common, caused by the long days of sitting and the usual ups and downs of life including concerns over jobs, family, and money. One of my favorite methods of bingeing was to have a bowl of cereal covered in sugar. I ate the first serving, then poured more cereal and more milk into the bowl, and of course more sugar. I ate bowl after bowl of cereal until I literally felt like I would pop. I did this alone, with no one around. Not even my husband was aware of my problem. I remember one day he said to me, "You don't eat very much, I don't know why you have trouble with your weight." I really didn't eat much in front of him, or anyone else. My overeating happened in private, when no one was around. That way I was able to mute my feelings of guilt and shame. Then it was just me and the food.

My severe binge eating phase lasted about 6 months, after which I was able to calm down a bit after listening to an Anthony Robbins tape where he explained how my bad habit was a protective mechanism I had created to protect myself from other things I perceived as being worse, in my case social anxiety. After this I resorted to just regular overeating, not the painful binge eating I had been stuck on. Unfortunately I still had a major obsession with sugar. I couldn't get enough of it. Sugar made me feel so good and I was not above eating straight spoonfuls of it just to get the sugar high.

In the years following, on work days I got in the habit of buying bags of candy at a local drug store close to my office. I smuggles the candy in to work with me and ate entire bags at my desk. I'm talking about entire bags here, not candy bars, and not a few pieces, but pounds and pounds of candy: anything chocolate, gummy everything, and anything else that sounded good for the day. I did this almost on a daily basis. In fact, I frequented the drug store so often that when I stopped eating all the candy and just went there to buy other items, the checkout clerks asked me if I was on a diet because I wasn't buying anything sweet. I was astounded at the question, and at the fact that more than one clerk knew my habits and asked me the same question on different days!

I can't entirely imagine the damage all that sugar did to my body, but it must have been pretty bad. I developed cavities at the age of 28, for the first time in my whole life. I never had problems with my teeth until this severe sugar-laden bingeing cycle. Also, at one point prior to starting the Leverage Diet, I was frequently taking an antibiotic, anti-inflammatory, anti-histamine, and anti-pain medicine all at the same time because I couldn't fight off infections like I used to. My immune system was tanking. My blood sugar swung violently every day. In the afternoons, the only way for me to remain half awake was to load up on more sugar.

I knew I was headed for some heavy duty problems if I didn't change my habits.

One of the final incidents I experienced in my overweight body happened at the copy machine at work. One day, while standing at the machine making copies, and I realized that the fat on my back was rolling up and putting so much pressure on my rib cage that I was having trouble breathing. I couldn't believe it. I thought to myself, how could I have let this happen? I have fat rolls and they are making it hard for me to breathe. I am a disaster. I can't keep living like this, I have to do something. Less than a month later I began my Leverage Diet.

Years of chronic dieting and emotional eating left me an overweight mess. But even though I had never been successful at controlling my eating or losing weight, and even though I still struggled with social anxiety, the Leverage Diet worked, and that's why I want to share it with you. If this method worked on someone like me, I have high hopes that it can help you too.

Chapter Two

The Leverage Diet

Lev-er-age: Leverage has several meanings, but the meaning I want to draw your attention to is "positional advantage, or the power to act effectively." (Wikipedia, 2011) Think about this: if you had the "power to act effectively" when it comes to losing weight, you could lose all the weight you want. Not only would you have the power, the means, and the ability, but you would use those things to act effectively and reach your goal. But here's the truth: you already have the power. You have the ability to make things happen in your life. You have the ability to take action and get from Point A to Point B. You already have the ability and the means to lose weight. How many times have you started a diet, and you did well on it for the first day or week or two, only to end up losing control and bingeing on whatever you could find? Then, you returned to your old eating habits, with no evidence that the diet you just tried ever happened. The question here is: why did you go off your diet plan? What made you lose control?

There is an honest truth about diets. Most nutritionists and diet experts out there would probably agree with me on this. The truth is, DIETS DO WORK! Why? Because diets are designed to cut out all those excess calories you eat so you can lose weight. Because our bodies function so that: we gain weight when we eat too many calories; we maintain weight when we eat just enough calories; and we lose weight when we don't eat enough calories. I'm sure you've heard this many times. Calories in have to be less than calories out, etc. etc. etc. It's true! Yes, there are some people with medical conditions that this does not apply to, and for that I am very sorry. But that is not a problem shared by the majority of people struggling to lose weight. Most people's bodies are going to follow the calorie rules.

We tend to make weight loss too complicated. We over-think the process and weave a tangled web of do-this-not-that requirements in order to lose weight. Atkins? Grapefruit Diet? How much protein? How many carbohydrates? How much fat? Should I do carbohydrate cycling? Which diet is the best diet? What about weight loss plateaus? Do weight loss pills work? How much exercise do I need?

The reason most of us are overweight in the first place is because we eat too much. Let me say that again: *The reason most of us are overweight in the first place is because we eat too much!* Whether over many years, or over a short period of time, we gain weight because we overeat. It's that simple. We all have different reasons for overeating, but the end result when we gain weight is caused by eating too much. Reversing our "overweight" problem takes no complicated action or special formula. All we have to do is endure a calorie deficit long enough for those extra pounds to fall off. Eat too many calories = gain weight. Eat a calorie deficit = lose weight. To lose weight we have to eat less, there is nothing complicated about that fact.

You may be worried that your metabolism will slow down so much that you won't lose weight on a lower calorie diet. But there's a misconception here that can prevent you from even trying to lose weight by eating less. The slowing metabolism issue is highly debated, and there are many factors involved. But in general, if you maintain a safe amount of calories during your diet, your body will hum along just fine as you drop the pounds.

Still not convinced that you need to eat less food in order to lose weight? Think about this: Do you really think that if you were stranded in the desert with no food for 30 days, that you would maintain your weight because your body would be in "starvation mode" and would't let go of any weight? I highly doubt that. Most likely, you would be very thin at the end of those 30 days if you were still alive, that is. Weight loss in itself is very simple. *The difficulty lies in sticking to a calorie deficit diet long enough to lose the weight.*

So now you're saying, ok, so how is this Leverage Diet going to be any different? The answer is simple: this isn't a diet; this is the *method* you are going to use to get yourself to *stick to* a diet! Oh, so you think you can stick to a diet by yourself, huh? Think again. If you're reading this, you've probably failed at every diet out there. How much money have you spent on diet shakes and pills, diet books, or pre-packaged diet foods? Ever buy exercise equipment from an infomercial that you only used once? Hmmm? Be honest with yourself.

I have tried just about every diet on the market. I have a graveyard of diets long past in my cupboards at home: half used bottles of diet pills, cartons of strawberry and chocolate diet shakes, and stacks upon stacks of those fun grocery isle magazines that advertise diets that say things like "The No more Belly Diet" or "The Be Skinny By Next Tuesday Diet". I even tried a weight loss patch when I was in high school. I thought I would just slap the patch on my arm and lose 20 pounds. And of course, that didn't happen.

If a mysterious money fairy suddenly appeared to show me a total of how much money I have spent out of desperation on diet books, pre-packaged meals, shakes, pills, patches, and the list goes on, I would probably pass out. Think about it: 15 years of dieting and buying oodles of diet foods/books/pills/packaged meals/shakes would cost enough money to have retired early. Ok, that's a bit of an exaggeration, but I confess that I have made a huge contribution to the multi-billion dollar diet industry.

The truth about those diets I tried is that they would have worked, if I had been able to stick to them. And no, I'm not trying to promote fad diets, or the diet product infomercials that guarantee you will look like a fitness model after 14 days and four installments of just $39.95. Many companies out there just want to make a sale. Once you buy their product, their venture has been a success. They use your emotions to get you to spend money. They know you really want to lose weight, so they present their material to you in a way that - by the time you are ready to buy that product - you are convinced that you are going to look like the fitness model in the infomercial as soon as you get it.

The purpose of this book is to give you a way to follow through with your wish to lose weight. You don't have to spend any more money on dieting, I promise. I mean, you can follow any of those diets out there – you probably have a dozen diet books still sitting around, right? So use them if you'd like. But you don't need to buy anything other than food to lose weight, which you would have to buy anyway just to stay alive!

The reason you failed all those diets for all these years, is because your desire and emotional need for too much food was stronger than your desire to lose weight. In fact, it was emotionally more comfortable not to be on a diet, since you probably use food for emotional balance. I know how it feels when you first start a diet and then begin to feel those initial hunger pangs. There is a bit of a panic that takes over, and you start thinking on a deep subconscious level, *I miss that food, that comfort, I don't think I can survive without it, I don't want to go through my whole day feeling empty!*

If you are like me, you are an emotional eater and you self-soothe with food on many different levels. You eat when you are happy: *Let's celebrate by going out to dinner!* You eat when you are stressed or angry: *This chocolate cake will make me feel better.* You eat when you are sad or lonely: *This donut is my friend and makes me happy!* Many studies have been done on emotional eating, and it's a tough one to crack because we are driven by our emotions in every aspect of our lives. It is hard for us to willingly submit ourselves to emotional discomfort or pain, so it is hard for people like you and me to give up those comfort foods and the urge to overeat because those things actually make us feel better.

The Leverage Diet short circuits the emotional overeating crisis by giving you the emotional Leverage to stay on a diet. It is so strong that you won't compromise. You can't take that risk. Again, when I say "stay on a diet", I mean eat less! If you don't already know how to cut back on calories, you may want to do some research first. There is a wealth of free information on the internet about cutting calories.

The basic idea is to *consume fewer calories consistently over time*. That's how you lose weight. You can follow one of those diet books you already have, if you'd like. The method of reducing your daily caloric input is up to you; just make sure you eat less than you burn. You don't even have to follow an exercise program to lose weight, even though I am a strong believer and supporter of the health and weight loss benefits of exercise. But if you don't have time or energy to exercise, you don't have to in order to lose weight. Just put less food in your mouth!

The following story is about how I discovered the emotional Leverage that finally got me to lose weight. I will tell you how I arrived at this Leverage that for me was immediately and 100% effective. In Chapter Three I will show you my actual weight loss data recorded in the process. And, you will find that I didn't radically change my lifestyle, all I did was eat less long enough to lose weight.

In October 2010, my husband and I attended a dinner event at a local country club. The event was also called a ghost hunt, and it was hosted by a local paranormal research group. The country club was several hundred years old, full of rich local history. We were served dinner and afterwards we were given a tour of the building and were told about the history of families and events that had taken place there.

The paranormal research group had us listen to several different tape recordings that captured paranormal voices in the facility. There were voices saying names or other strange phrases. We were also told about the strange occurrences that happened (and still happen today) that led them to believe the entire place is "haunted" by the remnants of humans long past. Today there are several ghost hunting reality shows on TV that show similar situations and studies as this one.

My husband may not admit it, but I think we both left there feeling a little green and scared out of our minds. We had never been exposed to anything like that before. Listening to the ghostly voices on tape was a complete and total shock. It was definitely one of the most mind-blowing and scary experiences I had ever encountered. I don't think we slept well for a few nights after that, especially after we realized that our own home was over a hundred years old and had the potential for some human remnants as well!

Now, this haunted country club had also been an inn for many years, and still is today. I thought to myself as we left that evening: I will never step foot in this place again. It is too scary, too real, and too much for me to handle. Unbeknownst to me at the time, that spine-tingling fear would become my weight loss Leverage.

A few weeks after our paranormal experience, the idea hit me like a bolt of lightning: I will make a bet with my husband that I will lose 20 pounds, or stay overnight by myself in that haunted inn. I was more than ready for the new challenge. I desperately wanted to find a way to literally *force* myself to lose weight, because I was tired of the overeating cycle and of the fact that my weight was directly tied to my self-esteem and self-confidence, dragging both lower and lower as my weight went higher and higher.

I was tired of having the first thought on my mind every morning upon waking be that of my weight. I was tired of having the final thought on my mind every evening before bed be that of my weight. My weight problem was like a torturous ball and chain that I dragged around every day for many years. It was a burden and a curse, and I didn't want it anymore.

I realized that I had to do something to lose those 20 pounds and to stop my fierce overeating habit. It wasn't fair to my husband. I knew he loved me even though I was heavier, but I also knew he would appreciate me being in better shape as the woman he married 5 years prior. And it wasn't fair to me; I never wanted to gain so much weight. An increase of 20 pounds on my 5'3-3/4" frame is nothing to laugh at. I didn't want my overeating to continue, and I didn't want to be unhealthy and self-conscious anymore.

So I made the bet with my husband: lose 20 pounds in 20 weeks, or stay at the haunted inn by myself. This Leverage was instantly enough to short circuit my emotional overeating habit. There was no way on earth I was going to set foot back in that haunted country club, especially not for a whole night by myself! The sheer terror that this invoked was enough to override my desire for all that sugary and fatty food. Fear of the haunted inn and of meeting ghosts alone in the dark became stronger than my need to overeat. It worked like a light switch.

My diet plan of attack was simple: I planned to eat between 1,200-1,500 calories a day through the week. I was stricter during the week days because I was on a schedule with work and it was easier to plan meals and meal times. I eased up slightly on weekends to between 1,500 and 1,800 calories, and one of those days I allowed myself to eat more than that. After 20 weeks of the self-imposed calorie deficit, I was sitting over 20 pounds lighter.

You probably think this is the juicy part of this book, where you look to see exactly what and when I ate, so you can do the same thing. But that's not the point! The point of this book is to get you to discover your Leverage, or the emotional scare tactic you are going to use to get yourself to stick to your diet. Once you find that, you'll be on the road to losing weight and feeling better.

Chapter Three

How To Find Your Leverage

If I were to offer you $20 million to lose 20 pounds, would you do it? I hope your answer is, *Heck, yes!* That would be my answer! Let's say you were a big time Hollywood actor/actress, and you were just hired to do a movie for a salary of $20 million. The producers told you that in order to fulfill the role you need to lose 20 pounds. Would you have any trouble skipping the double cheeseburgers at the drive-thru and instead eat less food until you lose the weight? I doubt you would have much trouble, with that kind of incentive waiting for you. I know I wouldn't!

Unfortunately, most of us don't have an offer like that on our table. As an emotional overeater, I've had a lot of trouble finding an incentive powerful enough to get me to stick to a diet and lose weight. Some women are able to lose weight for their wedding or other social gathering they are looking forward to, and they find that to be enough of an incentive to stick to a diet. But for the rest of us emotional overeaters, we may start a diet with the intention of losing weight for that wedding or reunion, but we quickly fall off the wagon and make the unconscious decision that the feelings of comfort and emotional fulfillment we get from placating ourselves with food is much more important than looking good at a party.

The basic principle here is for you to do some creative thinking and find a scenario or event that would force you into sticking to a diet and overpower your desire to keep overeating. Remember - my Leverage was the fear of having to spend the night in a haunted inn. There was no way I could handle going back there, so I did exactly what it took to lose those

20 pounds in those 20 weeks. I won the bet, lost the weight, and avoided the terror, all in one! Leverage is what will get you to stick to a diet long enough to lose that weight.

I stress to you that your Leverage should be more along the lines of facing the "stick" rather than winning the "carrot". Meaning, choose a punishment that you will avoid at all costs (i.e. you WILL follow a diet to avoid it!). If you have repeatedly failed all previous attempts at losing weight, don't you think it's time to try something different?

I realize that not everyone likes the idea or agrees that negative reinforcement works better than positive reinforcement. But in this case it really can! And IT WORKED FOR ME! And just who am I? I'm a regular woman that has struggled with body image issues and nearly life-long weight issues. I juggle jobs, a home to take care of, bills to pay, husband and family to love and take care of, social anxiety, and I am an emotional overeater and chronic dieter that has been 100% unsuccessful on every other approach to dieting except this one. This method worked for me, and I think it will work for many other women and men just like me.

Losing weight for the health and longevity benefits should be a good enough reason to do it, but unfortunately it isn't for many people. Let's momentarily look at being overweight from the scare-tactic side: if you don't lose weight and clean up your eating habits, you could get a disease or die early. That sounds pretty scary to me, but like I said, it just doesn't hit home for many people that are entrenched in their self-soothing habits of overeating.

I want to caution you that when you are searching for your Leverage, be sure it is safe, healthy, legal, and will not harm yourself or anyone else. That's my disclaimer. Use common sense, be safe to yourself and to others, and never put yourself or others in danger, whether physical or emotional.

Here are some samples of Leverage scare tactics that may help you come up with some ideas:

<u>Example 1</u>: I will lose 10 pounds in 10 weeks, or I will go sky diving with Ralph and Susie who are always trying to get me to go but I am way too scared ever to do.

<u>Example 2:</u> If I don't lose 15 pounds by May 1st, I will be seen in my swim suit at the local pool (which completely terrifies me).

<u>Example 3:</u> If I don't lose 15 pounds by May 1st, I will not get to go on our family vacation to Hawaii.

<u>Example 4</u>: I will ride the Rollercoaster From Hell at the local theme park 5 times if I don't lose 10 pounds by April 5th.

<u>Example 5:</u> I will stand in the center of town holding a sign that says "I can't follow a diet" if I don't lose 30 pounds in 3 months.

<u>Example 6</u>: If I don't lose 15 pounds in 15 weeks, I will dye my hair black (unless your hair is already black of course!) and wear it like that for 15 weeks.

<u>Example 7:</u> I will write a check to my friend for $500. If I don't lose the 20 pounds in 20 weeks my friend will

get to cash the check and I will lose $500 which I can't stand the idea of!

Do you get the idea? Your Leverage needs to be very powerful, yet still safe and healthy. It should be something personal to you, something that only you know just how horrible it would be to have to face the punishment for not following through on your commitment. That's exactly what the Leverage Diet is designed for, to get you to:

1. Stick to a diet plan
2. Lose the weight
3. Celebrate your success OR face the consequences if you don't fulfill your commitment

You need to be accountable not only for your commitment to the diet and losing weight, but for your commitment to the consequences if you don't lose the weight. Give yourself enough time to lose the weight (common sense goes here.) For example, plan to lose one pound a week for so many weeks. If you consistently follow the diet (in other words, eat less calories,) you will lose the weight, it's that simple. Your past dieting failures are due to the fact that you didn't have a strong enough, emotionally-charged reason to stick to the diet. But now, with Leverage, you do.

The other key to the Leverage Diet is that, once you find your Leverage, you need to make it known to someone or a group of friends that will help hold you to your goal. I made my bet with my husband. Of all the people I know, he is the one person that would hold my nose to the fire if that's what needs to happen. He is a no-nonsense, hold-you-accountable kind of guy. There's nothing wishy-washy or sugar-coated about him. He showed no weakness and no mercy. YOU need to find that kind of person, or group of people, and make your deal with them. Make your goal and your commitment known. Draw up a contract, sign it, and have someone else sign it as your witness, to make things interesting. This is exactly what I did. I wrote and signed a contract with my husband. Find someone that will hold you accountable to your plan. Find someone that will not show you mercy, if you don't follow through.

So first find your Leverage, the "punishment" that you will face if you don't fulfill your commitment. Then, get your Leverage witnessed by someone that will help you enforce it. During my weight loss phase, my husband would often say things like, "I already booked your room at the haunted inn!" or "You'll have to take some pictures of all the ghosts you're going to see when you stay at the inn by yourself!" Things like that only made my drive to lose the weight stronger, and made my fear of sleeping at the haunted inn that much more intense. Thanks to those comments, my commitment was strengthened. Behold the power of the stick!

Do you understand that my fear of staying at the haunted inn was stronger than my urge to comfort myself with food? Yes there were plenty of days where I *felt* like stuffing my belly with sugary and fatty foods, but I didn't. Plenty of days where the long work day was stressful, or I was tired, or there were just the normal ups and downs of everyday life that normally I would have chosen to soothe myself with something fried or fatty. And let's not forget about the ugly beast that rears its head for some women on a monthly basis: yep, I'm talking about premenstrual syndrome (PMS). With this I normally get fierce food cravings that are completely out of control and I habitually binge eat because of it. But the fear of losing the bet was stronger than the urge to comfort myself with food. Amazingly, t*he cycle of emotional overeating had effectively been destroyed and the Leverage had become an effective distraction technique.*

You will need to identify your specific Leverage. What are you so scared of, you will avoid at all costs? Then find the right person or group to help hold you to it. These things will give you that positional advantage, and help you use your innate power to act effectively and finally lose weight.

You may be wondering, what will happen if you don't meet your goal? The answer is simple. Take your medicine! Face the consequences! If you follow this program correctly, you commit to your goal, you secure Leverage over your emotions, and you recruit someone or some method to help hold you accountable. You not only commit to losing the weight, but you commit to the punishment that awaits you if you don't stick to the diet. So now it is time to be a person of integrity, of commitment, and of accountability. You may feel let down if you meet your goal, but it also may be an indication that you didn't choose the right kind of Leverage to begin with. And if that's the case, try it again, this time with the right kind of Leverage.

Chapter Four

Case Study: Real Data from the Leverage Diet

This is where I share with you the actual data I recorded from myself on the Leverage Diet. The steps I took were simple yet powerfully effective. From start to finish, here's the real data.

1. I made the bet with my husband: if I didn't lose 20 pounds within 20 weeks, I would stay overnight at the haunted inn by myself. I wrote this down on paper, signed, and dated it, and hung it up on a mirror in our bedroom as a consistent reminder.

2. I planned my diet: I chose to stick with a 1200-1500 calorie per day diet on work days. I packed my

lunches on weekdays and bought what I needed for meals each weekend when I went grocery shopping. Now, my eyes nearly cross whenever I read a diet book with recipes, and I don't have the time or mental energy to read a recipe, much less follow one for all of my meals. Between my daily commute and hours spent on the job, my work days are 12 hours long, after which I'm exhausted. So, microwaveable and frozen meals worked best for me. Here is a general idea of what my weekday meals were:

Breakfast: Yogurt, banana, or breakfast sandwich and tea.

Lunch: Soup or frozen meal (like Smart Ones, Healthy Choice, etc), cheese stick, grapes/orange/apple

Dinner: Frozen vegetables & grilled chicken made at home, or cereal & fruit.

Drinks: hot tea, iced tea, diet sodas

Snacks: fruits or raw vegetables, wheat crackers, chocolate.

One day a week I would allow myself to eat a "normal" meal that may have included something fried and a Coke to drink. I think doing this once-a-week routine helped keep my metabolism high and satisfied any cravings that may have popped up.

3. I followed my diet. During this time period I encountered holiday meals, birthday cakes, and cookies and snacks at work, all of which I partook in. Whenever I ate something in this category, I simply adjusted the food I ate the rest of the day so that the overall daily calories balanced out. So yes, I occasionally ate some chocolate, cake, candy, donuts, and other typical no-no's on this diet, and still lost weight, because I made sure to balance out any calorie "overages" the next day or two. It's that simple!

4. I began my diet weighing 175.8 pounds, and ended it weighing 153.3 pounds. I met my 20 pound loss goal at week 18.

5. I avoided the punishment. No haunted inns for me. I dodged the bullet! I escaped the stick! I fulfilled my commitment and lost the weight. Not only did I avoid the stick, I am now relishing my new figure and the confidence that has come along with finally losing

those 20 pounds that I used to think in desperation, would never come off.

6. The chart on the following page represents my actual data as shown in this table. I weighed myself once a week, every Monday at 6:30pm right before dinner:

Week	Date	Weight (lbs)
Start of Diet	1-Nov-10	175.8
Week 1	8-Nov-10	173.2
Week 2	15-Nov-10	173.8
Week 3	22-Nov-10	170.6
Week 4	29-Nov-10	169
Week 5	6-Dec-10	168
Week 6	13-Dec-10	167.1
Week 7	20-Dec-10	166
Week 8	27-Dec-10	165.5
Week 9	3-Jan-11	165
Week 10	10-Jan-11	164
Week 11	17-Jan-11	164.1
Week 12	24-Jan-11	163.2
Week 13	31-Jan-11	162.5
Week 14	7-Feb-11	161.3
Week 15	14-Feb-11	159.4
Week 16	21-Feb-11	157
Week 17	28-Feb-11	156.1
Week 18	7-Mar-11	155.8
Week 19	14-Mar-11	153.3
Week 20	21-Mar-11	153.3

As you can see, my weight loss was not fast. There were some weeks that showed a larger loss than others. Since I gave myself 20 weeks to lose the 20 pounds, I had to average out at 1 pound lost per week. So, those weeks in which I didn't lose a whole pound were made up in the weeks when I lost more than a pound. The rule of average calorie consumption played true here. I was able to enjoy the holidays and although I didn't lose much weight during the weeks surrounding Thanksgiving and Christmas, I was able to make up for that with other weeks.

The magic of this process is that not only did it work, but I didn't have to starve myself to lose the weight. I didn't have to eat lettuce soup for 20 weeks, or cut out carbohydrates. I simply followed the reduced calorie theory and it worked perfectly.

When I finished this book, I was more than 6 months past the completion of my Leverage Diet. During that time I successfully maintained my 20 pound weight loss. You may be wondering how I did that. As a result of the weight loss, I no longer felt the daily agony of being overweight, and I did not have the desire or the need to overeat to soothe myself. There were plenty of times when I did eat sugary or other not so healthy foods for comfort, but the difference was that I didn't *overeat* them. I wasn't stuck in the cycle anymore, and I didn't have a reason to keep perpetuating the bad behavior.

And, I was so happy with my new weight that I didn't want to ruin it by willingly going back to my overeating cycle. So, it was actually quite simple to maintain my weight. I continued to weight myself weekly, and if a pound or two began creeping up on me, I adjusted my calorie intake for the next week to get rid of it. I was surprised at how easy it was to maintain the new weight, and how the experience of finally losing those 20 pounds completely changed my emotional response to food. I was finally able to see just how strong of a hold emotional overeating had on me for all those years.

Chapter Five

Ghost Fat

After my Leverage Diet was over, and I was a successful 20+ pounds lighter, I ran into an interesting "problem" that I want you to be aware of. I call it Ghost Fat. You see, while I was losing weight, and as the scale gradually showed smaller numbers, a part of me didn't believe it was actually real. I recorded the data, and checked the numbers frequently to verify that I was indeed losing weight. But I just couldn't believe it was working.

Even my own eyes didn't believe I was thinner. When I looked at my reflection in the mirror, or in store front windows on the way in, I felt like something was terribly off. I felt like the mirrors and glass were lying to me, and that I should appear much larger than I did. It was haunting at first, which is why I named this phenomenon Ghost Fat.

Perhaps the biggest indicator of my successful weight loss was that my clothes became too big for me. I continued to wear the same clothes during the diet period, and when I reached the 20 pound weight loss goal, I had no choice but to go to the store and buy new clothes – two sizes smaller than I had been wearing for years.

I remember the day very well: my mother and I went to a department store to do some shopping. I picked out clothes in my regular size 14 and XL's and headed to the dressing room. I tried the clothes on, and they were way too big. Puzzled, I began searching for clothes of smaller sizes. I was almost starting to believe that I had indeed lost weight, but I wasn't convinced of it yet. I grabbed some size 10 clothing and went back to the dressing room. I was skeptical, and was on the verge of laughing at myself for thinking I could fit into a size 10. But then it happened. Not one piece of clothing, not two, but every single piece of clothing I picked out fit me wonderfully. Some were size 10's, some were mediums as opposed to the "extra large" I had been accustomed to for all these years. But all of them fit, every last beautiful one.

The reality of my weight loss had finally set in. Beethoven's Ode to Joy began playing so loud in my head that I was certain that the other women in the dressing room could hear it spilling out of my ears. If you've never heard this song, to me it's the most beautiful, victorious song ever created. It was loud and powerful, and it filled my soul with joyous feelings of elation. Colorful fireworks exploded victoriously in the eyes of my imagination. I could literally almost see the red blues, and yellows streaking through the sky, lighting up my entire world.

After the elation subsided, I paused to take several deep breaths to calm myself down. I wiped the tears of joy from my eyes. I took another brief moment to enjoy what had just happened, and then lovingly collected the clothes that fit me to perfection and exited the dressing room. I felt like I was floating on air, like I had been re-created as a more confident and beautiful version of myself.

The dressing room incident was a powerful affirmation that I had indeed lost the weight, but the feelings of Ghost Fat followed me around for a few months after the diet plan was over. They gradually lessened, but were very intense at first. So here are some suggesting for you on how to handle your own feelings of Ghost Fat once you have lost the weight:

1. Reassure yourself often that you did lose weight, that you do look thinner, and that your feelings of doubt and bewilderment are normal.

2. Look back at the data you kept as you recorded your weight loss numbers. Continue to weigh yourself

at least once a week so that you get affirmations that you are still at the lower weight.

3. Do not be upset if you gain a few pounds after you have completed your Leverage Diet. Give yourself a weight range to stay within. For example, if your target weight is 150, give yourself leniency to be between 150-155 pounds, and if you go over 155, go on weight maintenance for a week or two until you get back to your target range. If needed, use more Leverage to get yourself back to your ideal weight range.

4. Realize that the heavy ball and chain of your weight problem has been released, and it will take some time to adjust to not having to worry about it anymore. The feelings of Ghost Fat will gradually diminish.

5. Look at your beautiful self in the mirror, smile and say "I did it!"

Chapter Six

Leverage Other Things

Emotional overeating was my biggest problem for many years. Because I know how difficult it was to try to kick the problem through traditional means, this brings me to the conclusion that using the same kind of emotional Leverage could probably help solve other similar habitual problems.

Some habits are bad for us. Obviously, overeating is one of them. Others may include smoking, excessive drinking, bingeing and purging, and other activities that put our health at risk. And as you know, it is difficult to break habits that we have had for so long. It is even more difficult to break those habits that we have instilled in ourselves to serve the purpose of fulfilling an emotional need. For example, for me, overeating brought comfort and reduced my feelings of stress. It also helped me hide from my own feelings of shame about my weight, which is ironic because the very habit that caused me to gain weight also soothed me about having gained the weight.

Perhaps smoking does the same for you, or drinking, or some other habit that you know you should stop doing, but it's just too hard to give up.

That's where Leverage comes in. Imagine if you made a deal with your entire family, all of your friends, and even your co-workers, that if you do not completely stop smoking within 3 months time, you agree to let them send you to prison for 10 years. Don't you think you would do *whatever it took* to stop smoking in 3 months? This is an extreme example, just like the $20 million offer to lose 20 pounds. But it's effective in illustrating that, with the right kind of emotional Leverage, you can kick any habit without much difficulty.

It doesn't have to be a habit that you are trying to stop, in order to use Leverage to your advantage. You can use it to get yourself to stop procrastinating. Some examples are cleaning out that messy garage that has years of junk piling up. Maybe you want to take a new class, or to make a career change, but you're afraid to try something new. Whatever the issue, you can use this Leverage program to make yourself stick to any kind of plan to reach your goals. Don't be afraid to create a powerful "stick" that will chase you towards your dream!

Chapter Seven

Conclusion

Remember these key Leverage Diet points:

1. Find your Leverage: the highly undesirable event or punishment you will carry out if you do not stick to your diet.

2. Identify your specific weight loss goal: Make it practical and don't try to become a 110 pound supermodel in the process. I suggest you give yourself enough time to lose a maximum of 2 pounds per week. Don't try to lose 20 pounds in 1 week, that's not healthy or practical!

3. Choose your diet: plan your reduced-calorie diet. Here you can follow any type of diet plan as long as it results in consistently consuming fewer calories than you have been at your current weight. I recommend staying between 1200-1500 calories for women, and 1500-1800 calories for men because those are the "safe" calorie minimums that should not cause any health implications. Choose the kind of foods you like and that you will eat every day.

4. Make your plan known to someone else or a support group that will help hold you to it. Sign a contract, create a blog, or even get a group together that will follow the Leverage process with you.

5. Initiate your plan and follow it. Frequently remind yourself of the Leverage that you are using. Put a reminder on your frig or dresser at home, or in your wallet so that you have frequent reminders of your plan. Take a picture of your current weight on the scale and set it as the wallpaper on your cell phone or computer.

6. Reap the rewards when you reach your goal! If you don't reach your goal, face your punishment!

As I mentioned previously, be sure that your Leverage is strong enough to be effective, yet still safe and healthy for anyone involved. It may take some time for you to come up with the right kind of Leverage, but keep brainstorming until you find the right kind of "stick" that will get you to stay on your diet.

I sincerely hope that I have effectively shared with you how I used the principle of using emotional Leverage to finally lose weight. If you can't stick to a diet, please put some serious consideration into trying this method, because as someone who has failed every other dieting method, this was an absolute success for me, and I hope it will be for you too. I wish you the best of luck.

I also hope that by showing you my personal data and sharing my personal story with you, I've provided you with even more motivation. It's not every day that a woman (especially a shy one at that) will share her weight or eating habits with *anyone*, let alone the public and all the potential readers of her story! My goal has been to be as transparent as possible so that you can see my struggles and identify with all I have gone through. I am so amazed that I was able to stop overeating and lose weight, that I just had to share this with you and as many people as I can reach.

I would love to get feedback from you when you use your Leverage program. Send an e-mail about yourself and your story to: leveragediet@gmail.com. Please feel free to visit my website for the latest news in Leverage and health at: www.leveragediet.com.

Let's make this the last time you ever have to go on a diet!

Rachel E. Short

Rachel E. Short lives in Hillsboro, Ohio, with her handsome gladiator of a husband Mick, beloved dogs Dozer, Poncho, Pitty, Blue, horses, and llamas.

On the website www.leveragediet.com, you will find Before & After photos of me showing my 20 pound weight difference. The "Before" picture was taken at my pre-Leverage Diet weight of 175 pounds in July of 2009. The "After" picture was taken at my post-Leverage Diet weight of 153 pounds in September 2011.

The outfit I'm wearing in the After photo is very significant. I hadn't been able to wear those black pants since I first met my husband in 2004. The white shirt was given to me for being a participant in the 2010 Cincinnati Flying Pig Half Marathon, which I completed along with my husband and friends. At the time of the Half Marathon, I couldn't fit into the shirt. Now I can. ☺